I0417631

# Nich's Health Guide
## for **Kids**

Nicholas Jay
Nikolai Pizarro

Copyright © 2012 Nicholas Jay and Nikolai Pizarro

All rights reserved.

To my great mom Nikolai and my bestie Titan.

# DISCLAIMERS

*My mom says we have to write this:*

These statements have not been approved by the FDA and are intended for informational purposes only.

# Introduction

My name is Nicholas. I'm 8 and this is my health guide for kids.

I learned all about health from my mom. She's a health consultant (that's kind of like having a sports coach but for your health). She helps people be healthy, lose weight, learn to grow food, and all kinds of things. She's also my homeschool teacher so I'm with her every day. This means I listen to her talk about health and watch documentaries and videos with her **all...the...time**!

When I was around 5, I started asking her to explain the things I would hear her teach her clients. The more I learned, the more wanting to be healthy made sense to me. Learning more about health made it easier to eat healthy even when my mom wasn't around because I knew what eating junk would do to my body. It also made me more frustrated when I would see adults giving unhealthy foods to children or when I would see children asking for foods that were bad for them. I was always wanting to tell people to STOP eating junk foods and eat good foods instead. It would hurt me (still does) to see people drinking energy drinks and sodas or getting fast foods.

My mom always tells me it's rude to tell people what to do or criticize their food when they are buying or eating it. "Everyone has to make their own choices," my mom says. And, I totally get that but I want people to be healthy.

One day when I was 7 and my mom was writing her book, I had an idea: *what if I wrote my own book? Then, people could read the book and hear what I had to say. That wouldn't be rude.* So my mom agreed to help me type my own health book in my own words. Weeks later, when I was watching Minecraft videos on Youtube, I asked her if my book could also have videos of me explaining things about health. She thought it was a great idea. And that's how this project got started.

My mom gave me a memo recorder and I recorded a lot of things on what's healthy and why it's important and some of the things my mom has taught me along the way about how my body works. My mom and I listened to the memos. They were ALOT of them. As we listened, my mom took notes on her computer, typed them up, and organized them.

*This is where it got interesting.* She had me read the notes and I would have to explain my points as clearly as I could. She would type them again and I would read them again and on and on it went until we were able to write each section. Finally, I had to give her some ideas on some pictures for the book. I also had to find an illustrator to make my ideas come to life. It felt really cool to hire someone to do something. I felt like a boss-grown up when I got to pick the illustrator and *hire* her.

Writing a book took longer and was harder than I ever thought. It made me appreciate authors a lot more.

Of course everything I write doesn't have to be for you to do exactly. But, hopefully this book helps you start to be more interested in learning about your health. I hope you like my work. I really want to make a big difference in the world and I believe this book is a start.

# You Eat for the Future

If you are reading this book, you are most likely a kid.
Have you ever asked a grown up why you have to learn how to read,
write, and do math or even why you have to go to school as a child?
I'm sure you have. The answer probably sounded something like this:

*"You have to go to school and learn to do those things so when you are
an adult you can make money, take care of yourself and your family, solve
problems, and get along with people. What you do as a child prepares you for
what you will have to do as an adult."*

**It's the same thing with eating healthy and
taking care of ourselves**. We have to eat
the right things NOW so we can prepare
our bodies for the future. You won't
always eat junk food and get sick right
away or eat healthy foods and feel good
right away. Sometimes you will but most
times, you are doing it for the future.

The same way you have to try to get
good grades and work
on your behavior to
have future                                    success, you
have to be good to              your body now to have future
health. If you                     neglect your grades, behavior, or
body's health now,              your future can be compromised.

When people ask us              "what do you want to be when you
grow up?" We usually say: *a doctor , business owner, lawyer, or even an artist*.
Those are great answers.  But, remember, that you also want to be a
healthy adult.  That too is what you want to be when you grow up
and it all starts with doing something NOW.

# What Love Looks Like

I've left the house a time or two without permission and when my mom found me, all I could see was the worry on her face. Yes, she was mad because I broke the rules but more than anything she was worried about my safety. One time, she was so upset she started crying as soon as she saw me. I felt terrible.

"I was just at my friend's house mom. I'm fine". I said.

I didn't know what the big deal was. My friend's house was just a few houses down. I knew exactly where I was. I tried explaining this to make her feel better. It didn't work.

"Nicholas, I didn't know where you were, if a stranger took you or if you were hurt. I looked for you. I called and got no answer. Don't you know I would be devastated if something ever happened to you?" She replied.

And when she said that, I understood. She loves me more than anything.

Another time, I was running in the house and ran right into the closet's edge. My head split open and there was blood everywhere. When I was screaming in pain, my mom wasn't mad about me running in the house even though I had broken a house rule. She wasn't even mad about the blood dirtying my clothes or the carpet! All my mom was worried about (and she was sooooooo worried) was about my safety.

We went to the hospital and I ended up getting 4 staples. In a couple of weeks, the staples came off and I was as good as new. I didn't even have a scar! But, what if something had happened to me that was *really* bad? My whole family would have been in pain.

These events helped me realize that when my mom tells me not to leave without permission or to walk inside the house, she's not telling me because she wants to boss me around, she is telling me to protect me. She loves me and she needs to know that I am and will be okay. Because if something bad happens to me, her world will change.

Our parents and other adults want us to avoid negative things because they don't want us to get in trouble or sick. They want us to be happy children and successful adults. That's really why our moms, dads, aunts, uncles, godparents, grandmas, and grandpas ask us to cross the street and look both ways, to wear our seat belts, not to talk to strangers, to bring our jackets on a cold day, and to brush our teeth at night so we don't get cavities. Sometimes their actions feel a little like nagging but all of it comes down to love. When people love us they do not want us to get hurt in any way. Not ever. **That's what love looks like.**

*Okay so…how is this about being healthy? Keep reading.*

I already told you that my mom and the adults in my life are constantly trying to keep me safe with their rules and their teachings, right? That is how they love ME.

But you want to know what I also learned? How I love them BACK is by loving myself and doing the things that protect and make me better.

I want to grow up and be a happy, kind, helpful, healthy person. I don't want negative things to happen to me. I'm still a kid so I make mistakes and forget to do the right thing all the time but, I try. I do these things because I am both loved and I love my family.

3

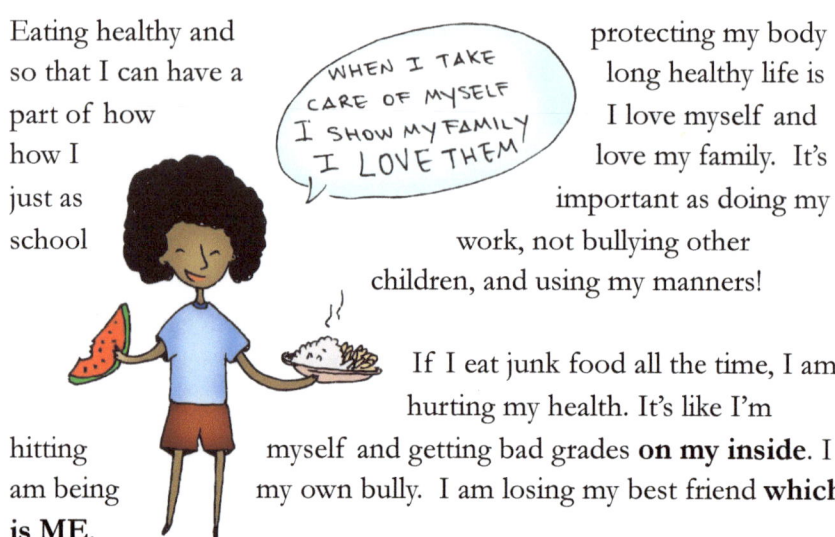

Eating healthy and protecting my body
so that I can have a long healthy life is
part of how I love myself and
how I love my family. It's
just as important as doing my
school work, not bullying other
children, and using my manners!

If I eat junk food all the time, I am
hurting my health. It's like I'm
hitting myself and getting bad grades **on my inside**. I
am being my own bully. I am losing my best friend **which
is ME**.

I am my family's treasure. They love me. I don't want them to hurt if something happens to me. I don't want to get sick. I want to have a strong body and mind that can accomplish anything.

Like me, you should chose to love yourself. Every time you say no to junk food and yes to a healthier food you should be happy and remind yourself that what you are doing is loving yourself *and your family.*

# WARNING

In this book, I will talk about eating healthy foods and not eating unhealthy foods ALOT because that's something most kids need to learn to do. But, before I do that I have to give you guys a big, big, BIG warning: **a lot of** **junk food tastes *delicious*!** In fact, the main problem with NOT eating unhealthy foods like donuts, brownies, cookies, hot dogs, burgers, and cheese puffs is that those foods taste reeeeeeaaaaaallllly good!

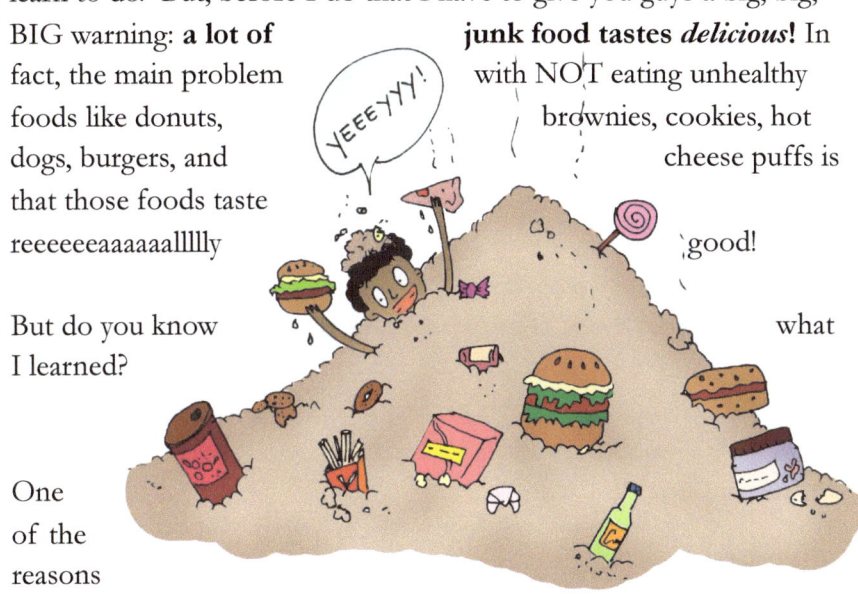

But do you know what I learned?

One of the reasons that those foods taste so good is because they have ingredients and chemicals that trick our brains and our taste buds. Some of those ingredients, like wheat and sugar, are also very addictive. Addictive means that you want more and more of something once you have it. Other ingredients such as MSG also make brains want more foods with chemicals in them. Because of these chemicals and ingredients, the more junk food you eat, the more you like it and the less you like and want healthy foods.

The people who make the foods are called food manufacturers. Food manufacturers don't care about the health of the people who eat their foods because they don't know them. They just care about selling more food because that's how they make money. The more food they sell, the more money they make. Of course they want to put chemicals and ingredients that make you want their foods!

Food manufacturers also know that kids don't read food labels and that we don't know that much about health. So on top of adding addictive ingredients and chemicals that make us want more of the junk food, they also spend a lot of money on commercials and packaging (the boxes and wrappers the foods come in) for fast foods and junk foods targeted at kids. They know that if they make the foods sound and look more exciting, kids will ask their parents to get them.

Next time you are watching anything on TV or online, count how many commercials there are for junk foods and fast foods. Notice how fun they make the foods and the packages on commercials or at the store. Food manufacturers don't care about your health at all, they just care about tricking you into wanting and liking their unhealthy foods, even if it will make you sick! Isn't that a horrible thing to do?

I really like the taste of junk food too so I understand that you will want them. Sometimes when I am at the grocery store and I walk by cakes and cookies I whine to my mom about how hard is it to be around all the delicious food and know that I really can't have them. Other times, I want pizza and candy sooooooo bad! I do. But, I think about the consequences that come with eating those foods like getting sick when I am older. I also think about those people making junk foods and get so angry with them. I do NOT like being tricked by people who think I don't know any better and don't care about hurting me. When I really want something junky, I think about these things and it makes me want it less.

Yes, junk food is tasty but it is..well…JUNK. I'm not a junky kid. I'm a healthy, strong, child that's smart. That's who I am. **You have to decide, who YOU are going to be. Your food defines you.**

# Healthy Body Basics

# Kids Should Know The Truth

When we started working on this book, my mom noticed I had a lot of memos about things like gut health, GMOs, and inflammation. You know, stuff that most kids don't talk about. She asked me if I really wanted to talk about those topics or if I just wanted to have a book that was more kid-like and fun. She explained to me:

> *"Some people, kids included, get a little scared when they think about diseases. The reason you hear and know so much about these things is because of the work I do. But, it may not be what kids really want to read about."*

I reminded her of the day I asked her why she had to teach grown ups about foods and how their bodies and diseases worked and she answered:

> *"Because no one teaches us these things when we are children and many of us grow up eating and doing things the wrong way our entire lives before we learn the truth. By then, a lot of us are sick or unhealthy. It would be so much easier if we just knew the right things from the beginning."*

So now that I was writing my own book that's what I wanted to do. I want to teach kids about health so we don't have to grow up our whole lives being unhealthy.

It's not that I want us to think about being sick all the time. We're kids. We shouldn't be worried or stressed with negative things like diseases. But, just like we should know the dangers of strangers and the consequences of doing the wrong things in life, we SHOULD know what happens when we are are not healthy. Children deserve to know the truth.

The more you understand how your body works and how important and fragile it is (that means it can get hurt easily) the more you will want to take care of it. The way you take care of it is mostly by eating good foods and not eating bad foods. I want you to know about your body and food because I care about you. Even if I don't know you, I still care about you.

These next sections of the book are all about different parts of our bodies and how food affects them. These are the things I have learned from listening to my mother and her clients and also by asking a lot of questions. I hope they motivate you to eat healthy like they have me.

## Mucus and Inflammation

In her work, my mom talks to her clients about inflammation and mucus A LOT. That's because when the body has excess inflammation and mucus for a long time it starts to get sick and feel pain. So, it's important to talk about them.

One day, I asked her to explain what mucus and inflammation were so I could understand why they were so bad for us. It turns out, inflammation and mucus are good for us but they can be bad also and that was a little confusing. Lucky for me, my mom has lots of patience and is really good at explaining health stuff.

She's going to write the next section and explain it to you exactly how she explained it to me.

*Hi I'm Nicholas' Mom. I'll take it from here.*

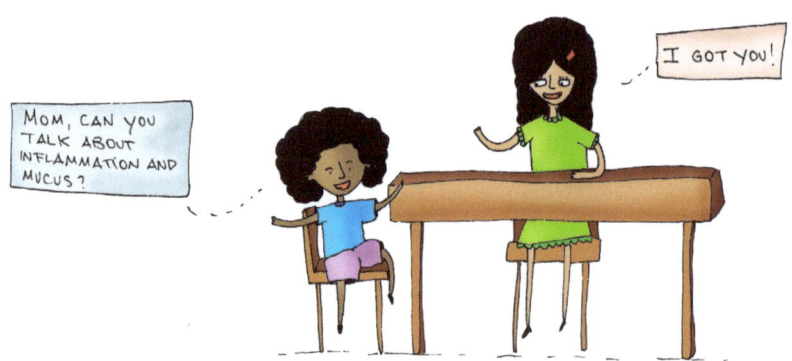

Many parents discuss negative situations with their children so that they can prepare for them in the event that they happen. Some examples might include things like bullying, a stranger approaching them, or a natural disaster like a storm, which can destroy their houses or shut off the power for days.

Faced with any of those situations, what are some of the things we could do? Some of the things Nicholas and I came up with were that he could walk away or find an adult that could help if he was being bullied. He could scream and run as fast as he could in case a stranger approached him. And, we could prepare a box in our home or car with flashlights, candles, firewood, a few days worth of food and water, or have a to-go backpack ready in case we need to leave our home in a hurry in the event of a storm.

I am sure these are some of the same things you too would think of doing. They are all the things that you could do to help yourself if you were in a pickle. Planning and preparing are defensive tools. They are ways to defend or protect ourselves from a negative situation.

Now that you understand what defensive tools are and how good it is to have them. I want you to think about what would happen if you had to use your defenses **every day** because **every day you** were in a dangerous or difficult situation. If that bully kept coming at you every single day? If it was more than one stranger and you were alone? What if you had to run for 20 minutes to safety daily? Or if the storm turned the power off for a month instead of a few days? At that point, your *tools* would give out because the situation was just too much to handle.

Defense plans and tools are usually things that can protect us for a short period of time. Being exposed to danger repeatedly or indefinitely, can change the outcome no matter how good a plan or tool is. And the absolute BEST way to protect ourselves against danger is to avoid it altogether if possible.

Think about it: what's safer? To face a bully and have a plan or not face one at all? Not being exposed to a negative situation is always a safer bet.

Now, let me tell you how this relates to your health.

Inflammation and mucus are our bodies defensive tools or *defense mechanisms*. When something like an infection or a splinter enters the body that's not supposed to be there, a whole army of helpers creates a protective shield around the area. Every little member of that army is working to help that area heal or at least not to spread to the rest of the body. That response is called inflammation. Inflammation contains the problem.

The same thing can be said about mucus. When you think of the word mucus, you can think of *snot!* Mucus is a type of wet, sticky stuff that's all over the back of our throats, mouths, nose, lungs, and other parts of our bodies, all the way to our gut. Mucus keeps everything moist inside us and catches germs and outside substances. It is another of our body's defense mechanisms.

If you can picture what happens when you have a splinter stuck in your finger, a sore throat, or a cold, you can envision how the whole area around that splinter, back of throat, or nose gets swollen and red. You'll also notice wet, slimy stuff that you have to cough up, blow out, or squeeze out of our finger. What you are seeing here are inflammation and mucus! Your defensive armies are rallying around the splinter or infection because those things aren't supposed to be there. Mucus and inflammation are containing the problem and protecting your body with a thick wall of puffy, slimy, sticky stuff. That's how inflammation and mucus are awesome. A normal amount of mucus is good to keep your lungs wet and your air flowing. A little inflammation helps you along the way.

The problem is that the body needs inflammation and mucus in the **right** amounts. When there is too much inflammation or when the body is having an inflammatory response all the time, it gets stressed out and tired. If you are constantly full of inflammation and mucus, you can end up very sick and feeling miserable.

Over short periods of time or emergencies, your body is good at defending itself. What your body is not good at doing is having to do that over and over again for a very long time. Too much inflammation and mucus in the body usually means that you are sick or on your way there.

A lot adults talk about having to reduce mucus and inflammation in order to cure diseases. But, inflammation and mucus are not the bad guys per say. Just like screaming, running, and the emergency food supply in your house are not bad things. The bad guys are the bullies, the storm, or the strangers trying to hurt you. What we need to to really do is stop the BAD GUYS and the BAD SITUATIONS! Because if we can stop THEM from coming into our bodies, then our bodies can stop producing excess mucus and inflammation.

What are those bad guys and situations and how do we get into them? Well, mostly food. The wrong foods can be inflammatory and cause our bodies to have excess mucus. It is the excess that doesn't let the body work properly. Our bodies simply can't function if they are swollen and full of extra mucus all the time.

There are a lot of adults that have diseases today because they have been eating foods that cause inflammation since they were little. After so many years of these conditions, their bodies break down.

Another bad guy's name is STRESS. Stress comes from not getting enough sleep, watching too much tv, not getting enough exercise, arguing, using harsh words, and worrying too much. Excess stress means excess mucus and inflammation.

There are foods and activities that reduce inflammation and mucus. They have opposite effect on our bodies.

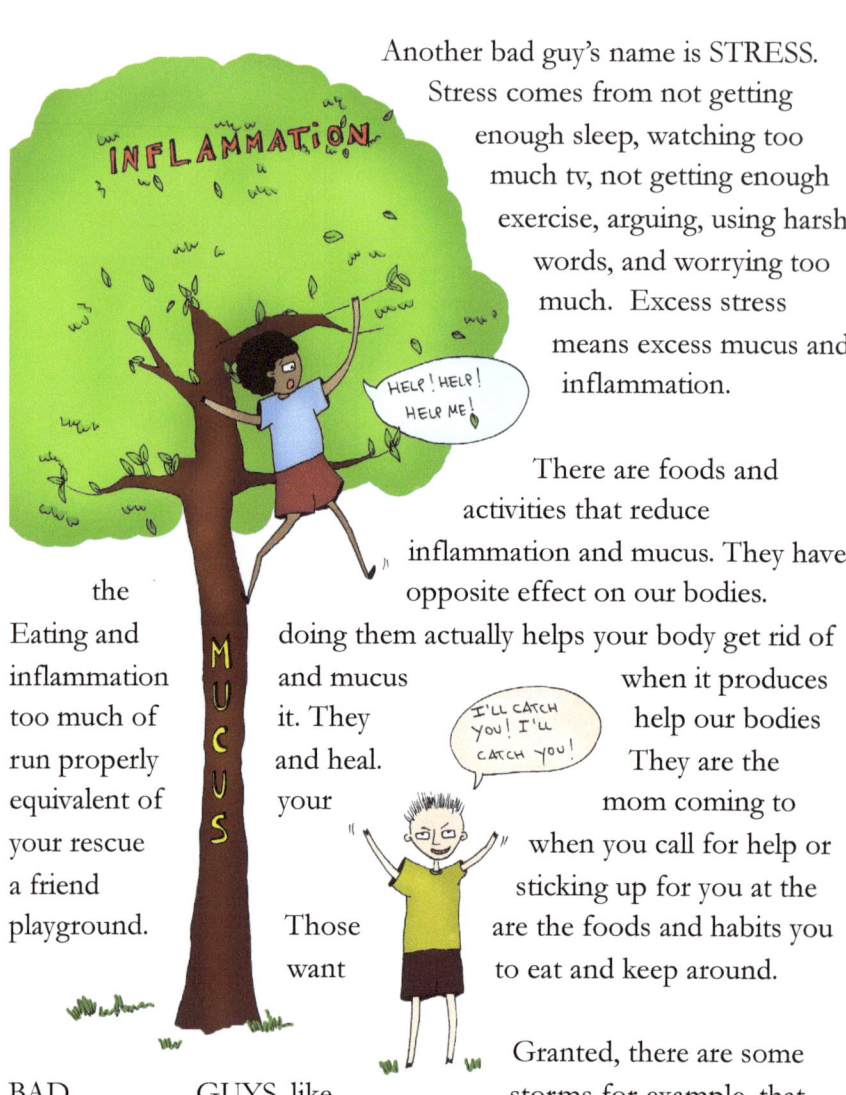

the
Eating and
inflammation
too much of
run properly
equivalent of
your rescue
a friend
playground.

doing them actually helps your body get rid of
and mucus                when it produces
it. They                help our bodies
and heal.                They are the
your                mom coming to
when you call for help or
sticking up for you at the
Those                are the foods and habits you
want                to eat and keep around.

BAD          GUYS, like          storms for example, that
we just have no control of. That's exactly why our bodies have built
in defense mechanisms. But, we should try our best to stay out of
harms way by making better choices in the areas that we can control.

Our job is to stay away from inflammatory, mucus producing foods
and stress (**avoid the bad guys)** and instead, get a good amount of
good foods and habits that reduce inflammation and mucus (**keep**

14

**the good guys)**. This is how we build ourselves up for when we do have to defend ourselves.

Your body is amazing and will do everything it can do to protect you from harm. But if you continually put it in threatening situations, it will get tired. You should learn what foods and things cause inflammation and mucus, remember them, and in the end eat less or avoid them. That's a TRUE defensive plan.

*Now, back to Nicholas.*

# Acid and Alkaline: The Kid Version

What I am about to tell you most grown ups don't know. *Actually, there is a lot of stuff in this book that a lot grown ups don't know. At some point, you'll have to catch them up.* Take your time and read this section slowly because this little bit of information can seriously keep you healthy for a long, long time.

There is this thing called a Ph scale. It's basically a number line and it measures things from acid to alkaline. The lower the number on the scale the more acid, the higher the number the more alkaline. *If you want to do a fun little experiment in the house, have your parents buy some ph strips and set out different liquids like tap water, bottled water, soda, apple juice, lemon water, and water with baking soda. Use the strips to measure how acid or alkaline each is and compare them.*

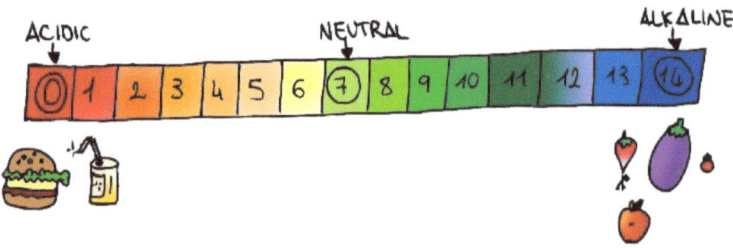

The inside of our bodies is supposed to be a little bit on the alkaline side and it turns out that there are certain diseases like cancer, *which is really, really bad*, don't like alkaline bodies. Diseases tend to like acidic bodies instead. This means that if you want to avoid or fight those diseases the best thing to do is to keep your body fairly alkaline. The trick is keeping your body in its balanced alkaline state. If you can do that, you can end up living a longer, healthier life.

Now, you know the whole thing about inflammation and mucus? Well, it turns out that most of the foods that keep your body acidic are the basically the same foods that also produce excess inflammation and mucus *annnnd* most of the foods that help your body be more alkaline are the same foods that fight them! This means that if you learn to do one, you usually end up with both. Pretty cool, huh?

Stay away from junk foods, processed foods, regular wheat, regular juices, sodas, sugar, and dairy. These products are usually packaged

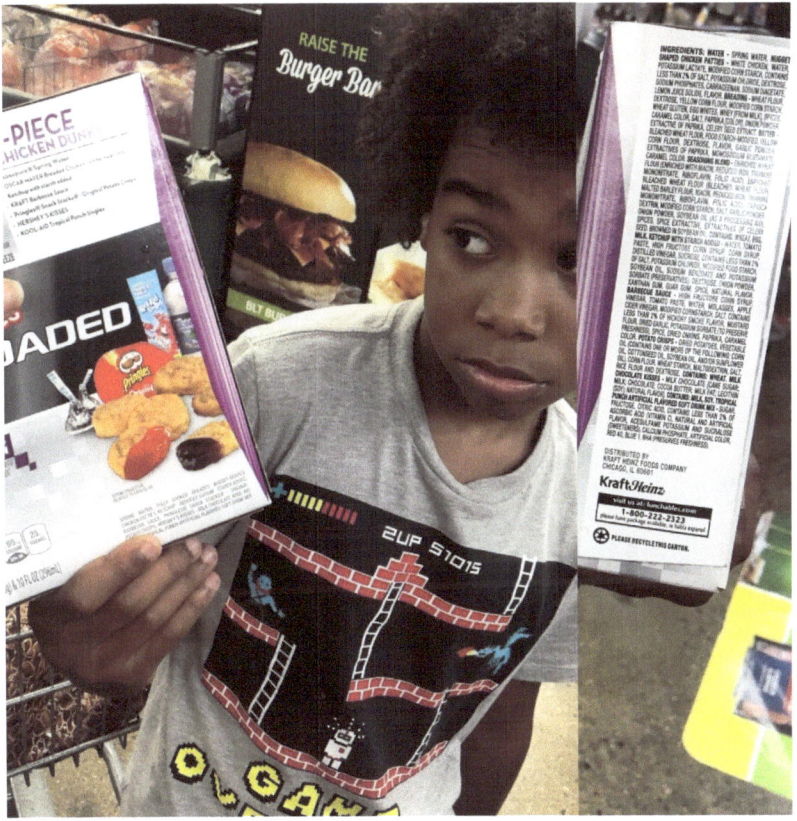

and have long lists of ingredients and toxic chemicals. Instead, eat more vegetables, fruits, and drink water. This will keep your body more alkaline **and** also reduce mucus and inflammation.

Not getting outside or sleeping enough and playing too many videos games or watching too much tv can also make your body acidic because they are all things that make our body more stressed. So, on top of not eating junk food and eating healthy foods and water, you need to try to get more time reading, resting, playing outside, laughing, and even meditating. These are winning, healthy habits.

# A Strong Large Brain

Your brain manages every thing that your body does. You don't just think with your brain. You move with your brain. You breathe with your brain. You eat with your brain. You laugh with your brain. A strong brain will help you learn quicker, control your body's impulses, fight disease…even run faster! You want to have the strongest brain possible if you want to be healthy. When the brain is weak, you forget things, you get sick, and you can have problems with your behavior.

Sugar and chemicals make your brain weak. Vegetables, fruits, and healthy fats make your brain strong. If you want a strong brain, don't eat lots of sugar and chemicals and also, eat lots of vegetables, fruits, and healthy fats. It's a no-brainer…*get it…no-brainer? Okay. That's supposed to be funny.*

But, seriously, your brain is responsible for memory, moods, feelings, and how you control your body. This means that when sugar and other chemicals affect it, we can have problems remembering, concentrating, controlling our bodies and a lot more. You will never be your strongest, best self if you are eating foods that weaken your brain.

I want to keep all my memories intact and be in control of my feelings and body. Don't you? I'm sure you do. So you have to avoid the wrong foods and eat the right foods…for brain's sake.

Did you know that sugar really does shrink your brain? It's true. Google "does sugar shrink your brain" and see all the articles that pop up. Read them with your parents and talk about them.

19

# Gut Matters

The body is like a machine. It needs all of its parts to work in order to run well. But, there are some parts that are bigger deals than others because without them, there is NO machine at all. Like your brain for example and your heart. We know those are BIIIIGGGG deals. You can live without you legs but you can't live without your heart or brain! Most of us know about the brain and the heart. But, there are other parts of the body that are super big deals too.

Did you know that there is one other organ in your body that's like your SECOND brain, it protects you all day long and no one ever really ever talks about it? *Well, except for if you live in my house because my mom sure talks* about it *all the time!* It's called your GUT.

The immune system is the system in your body that protects you from disease. When people talk about your immune system being weak or strong, they are really talking about your gut.

When you start to feel like you are getting sick and get a fever and your belly or head hurts and you want to sleep, what you are really feeling is your body fighting a battle. It is YOUR immune system fighting a virus or bacteria (the stuff that makes you sick).

Where is that battle happening? Mostly, in your gut! Your body's army lives there. It is full of good bacteria that fights back bad bacteria.

And guess what? Good bacteria, the kind that fights for you likes healthy foods. It is also very sensitive to certain foods like wheat, chemicals, and sugar.

Bad bacteria loves junk food. When the bad bacteria takes over, parasites, yeast, and other organisms (creepy critters and yucky beings) come live in your gut. Those guys need to eat to stay alive. They steal your nutrients and they start sending your brains signals to feed it. But, since they don't like health food, they start ordering junk food and you start craving and wanting to eat MORE sugar, more junk food, more wheat, and more chemicals because that's what *they* like to eat. It's like they take over your brain!

As you eat the junk food that you crave, you are feeding those creepy organisms and making them stronger. You are also making the GOOD bacteria weaker, *specially if you don't eat lots of healthy foods like vegetables.* Weaker good bacteria means that you start to create excess inflammation and mucus in your gut. Over time, you can even cause your gut to get so weak, it leaks!

Eventually, your good bacteria will be too weak to fight and the nutrients that your gut is supposed to keep in will get out. You can get asthma, allergies, eczema, itchy skin, behavior problems, ear infections, and other serious diseases once your army is sick. You don't want that. You need to protect your gut and give it good foods that keep it strong so that it can protect YOU.

How do you protect your gut? By not eating bad foods and eating lots of good health foods and since your gut is your second brain, *this is also a no-brainer.* Get it?!

Whenever you are eating, start asking yourself, am I feeding good bacteria or bad bacteria? Am I taking care of my gut so it can protect me or am I being careless and making it weak?

## Your Clean Up Crew

Inside of your body you have a clean up crew. These are the parts of your body that clean your blood so that junk and waste doesn't travel through your body and poison you. Your body is very sensitive. If your blood isn't clean and toxins are released into your body you can get very, very sick.

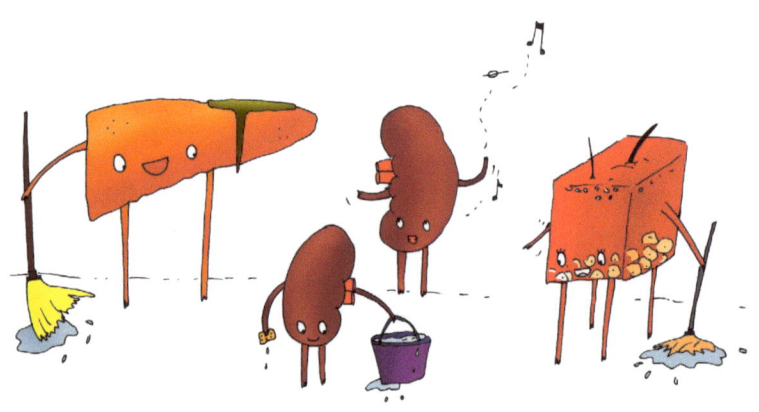

Your body gets rid of waste 3 ways. There is urine (pee), stool (poop), and sweat. Your kidneys make urine, your stools are passed through your intestines, and you already know, your sweat comes out of your skin. *Kidneys, intestines, and skin* are all parts of your cleaning crew.

**Your liver** is a another part of the cleaning crew. It is actually one of the most important members of the clean up crew because detoxifies (that's a big word for gets rid of) toxins OUT of the blood and keeps the nutrients IN the blood. Your liver can also save good nutrients that you don't need now for later when you do need them (kind of like packing a snack for you). If you want clean healthy blood, then your liver is your dude.

You have two **kidneys.** They are also blood filters but they do different things than the liver. Without your kidneys, waste builds up in the blood and damages your body. But your kidneys don't just filter your blood. Your kidneys also help your blood keep the right amount of water and nutrients in your body. This balance is what helps your body's blood flow, bones grow, and keeps your body hydrated. When your kidneys aren't working then your organs aren't hydrated and your blood can't flow right and your bones can't stay strong. This can make your heart and brain STOP and lots other painful things. You **definitely** don't want that to happen.

Your **intestines (a part of your gut)** is where your stool starts to form and you already know how dirty stool is. Your stool is all the waste and gunk that your body does NOT need. If you have the right amount of fiber and water going through the intestine and if your intestines are healthy then your body gets get rid of waste easily and your system is nice and clean. This is what keeps us healthy. Good fiber is found in mostly in vegetables and fruits. That's one of the reasons it's so important to eat them. If your intestines have inflammation and mucus and you don't have water and fiber in your system then, the waste stays in your body and can even go back into your bloodstream! Dirty toxic blood in your body? That's NOT good. You get sick that way.

The final member of your clean up crew is your **skin**. Your skin covers your entire body, from your head to your toes. So, your skin is really your **PROTECTIVE SHIELD** from the world. Your liver and kidneys are your INSIDE filters and your skin is your OUTSIDE filter. Your skin keeps toxins from getting IN your body and also gets toxins OUT using your sweat. You know how sometimes sweat smells and tastes funny? Those are your toxins getting out and your salts and water staying in balance. Keeping your skin healthy and clean and drinking water so that the skin can do its job is very important.

23

Now that you know that you have a clean up crew, I want you to imagine something that will help you understand what happens when you eat junk or processed foods often (or every day).

Picture your mom telling you that in order to go out and play with your friends, toys, or video games, **you first had to clean your room.** Imagine that you were motivated and you did a really good job and cleaned everything up so you could go play and as you were finished cleaning up your room, your little brother or sister came behind you and messed the whole room up again so, you cleaned it again. As your mom was coming to check it out, your little brother

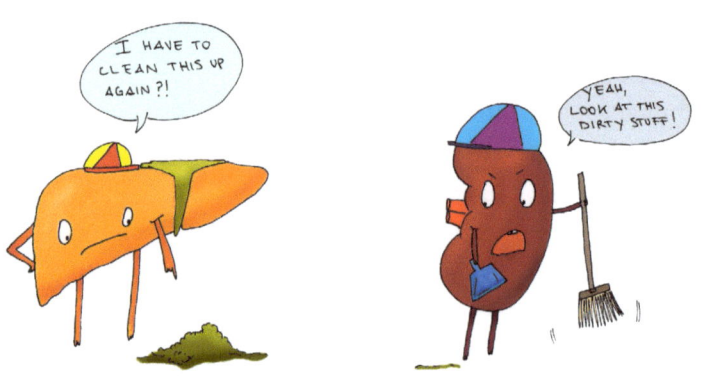

or sister came in and messed it up even worse! And your mom said to clean it up again.

Imagined that this happened over and over again. At some point, you no matter how badly you wanted to go outside and play, you would get tired, it would be time to go to bed, and you would feel defeated. If this happened every single day, you would not want to clean up any more. Even thinking of going outside to play wouldn't be motivating enough if you knew that every time your cleaning efforts would be in vain. That's how your liver, kidneys, intestines and skin feel over time if we eat the junkiest of foods every single day!

Most of us were born with a healthy clean up crew that's ready to work for us and keep us healthy. But, eating unhealthy foods is like constantly dirtying our system and making our crew work extra hard all the time. Over time, that clean up crew gets worn out and sometimes it quits on us. Without a clean up crew you have a dirty body that can't work properly.

We all have the power to keep our bodies working by taking care of it. Take it easy on the clean up crew, these guys are working for you. Don't eat food that work them overtime every day. They need a break too.

---

You know what your skin looks like. You see it every day. But do you know that your skin also made up of layers all of which you can't see? Find out what your skin really looks like underneath all the layers using the internet.

And while you are at it, research what your liver and kidneys look like too!

The more you learn about your body and its functions, the more you will learn to appreciate it.

---

# Pancre-WHO?

You probably never think about your pancreas. I know I never used to. But we all need a healthy, happy pancreas. Your pancreas is your friend. And, when your pancreas is sad, tired, and sick, it makes a whole lot of other parts of your body sad, tired, and sick also.

In order for you to understand why the pancreas is so important, you have to learn a little bit about *hormones* and what they do. Your organs (individual parts) do a lot of things. Your brain learns, your heart pumps, your stomach digests, and so on. But, in order for them to do those things, they need *hormones*.

Hormones are fuel. The parts of a car make it run but, it needs gas, oil, and water to actually do anything. Gas, oil, and water are the hormones of the car. Your XBOX controller can send signals to the console so you can play your games but, it needs batteries to do it. The console can play the games but, it needs to be plugged up to the wall. Batteries are the hormones of the controller. Electricity is the hormones of the console. How useful is a car without gas? A controller without batteries? A console if it's not plugged up? Not very. How useful are organs without hormones? Not very.

The parts of the body that make hormones are called glands. And that guys, is why the pancreas is so SUPER important. The pancreas is a major gland. It's another reason why its friend the liver is also so important. The liver, proud member of your clean up crew, is another major gland. You may not have heard of them until today, but glands are vital. You WANT to take care of them!

**Back to your pancreas.** Most of the food we eat is broken down into sugar and used as energy. Our bodies need energy to run on as its fuel. The most important thing your pancreas does is that it makes the hormones and enzymes that help your body break down and

26

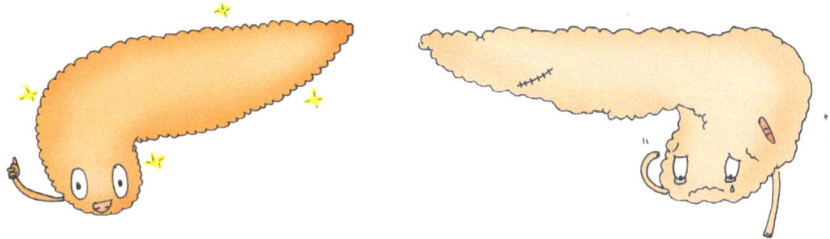

manage the sugar in the foods you eat.  If your pancreas is not healthy then your sugar levels are not balanced.

Think a car's gas tank for a minute. If you try to over fill it, gas spills out and if the tank is empty, the car stops. Our bodies are just like that. Balance is what your body needs so things can work right.  If your body can't break down and balance sugar, you have too much of it in your system at once.  This makes your blood vessels (what carries your blood through your body) get hard like candy shells and that makes your heart and brain stop working. **TRAGGGGGIC!**  Too little sugar or fuel is also tragic. It means you don't have enough fuel in your body and can't function.

There are lots of cool videos on Youtube that will teach you a lot of about how your organs and how health work. Here is a great one to learn about the pancreas.

Youtube: **What does the pancreas do? - Emma Bryce**

What are some of the things that can happen if your pancreas is not working and your sugar is not balanced?

Well, for one, your kidneys can become overwhelmed with too much sugar to filter. Over time this will make your kidneys shut down. Remember, your kidneys are a part of your clean up crew.  If your kidneys shut down they can't keep your blood clean or your water and nutrients levels balanced. Since, the clean up crew must all work together, when the kidneys are not working right, other crew members, like the liver get overworked and shut down also. This means more toxins in the blood, less glands working, less hormones to keep organs going, less hydration in the body…**everything starts to crash!**

And there is more…

When sugar levels aren't balanced, the hormones that manage stress are also out of whack. Remember what happens when you have too much stress? Your body builds up its defenses: mucus and inflammation and too much of that does what? Make you sick! Are you beginning to see how it's all super connected? When one thing isn't working, everything is affected and over time, your whole body can get really, really sick. So while you are not thinking of your pancreas, your pancreas is certainly thinking *and* working for you. If it shuts down, you are in big trouble. You want a happy pancreas.

How do we damage the pancreas? By eating junky, sugary, toxic foods and being stressed out. How do we help it? I'll let you guess. It's the same formula that keeps our body alkaline, reduces inflammation and mucus, makes our brain and gut strong, and keeps our clean up crew rested. Yup! We help it by eating vegetables, fruits, drinking water, resting, and exercising. It's that easy.

> Don't you feel good already knowing that you are protecting yourself by learning what to do early? I know I do.

28

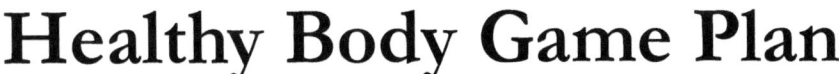

# Healthy Body Game Plan

# What's Next?

I have shared most of what I know about keeping a healthy body so far and why it is important. I hope you have learned that there are a lot of things going on inside your body that can shut down by eating the wrong foods and not eating the right foods and that you understand that taking care of your health is a way to love yourself and your family. I also hope you understand the things you eat and drink today as child will affect you as a grown up.

Before I knew about how my body worked and my mom would just tell me to eat healthy, I would    get frustrated. I just wanted the yummy foods my friends had **not** the healthy foods my mom    was giving me all the time. But, once I started to really    understand how it was all connected, making healthy decisions got easier. Hopefully, you are starting feel the same way.

Now that you know a little, *well a lot really*, about how good and bad foods affect your body, let's talk about what to eat, what to do, and how to do it.

## It's Better With Friends

You know how playing Minecraft or Legos or whatever it is that you are into is better with friends? Having a healthy lifestyle is the same way. It's easier to do things when your friends and your family are doing them also.

One of the reasons it's easy for me to eat the way that I do is because my mom eats and lives this way and a lot of her friends and her friend's children (who are also my friends) do too.

We all have to learn and work together. So as you read this book and learn some of these tips and concepts, think about your friends and family and share the information with them. Try new healthy foods and look through the ingredients of the things you are eating together. Go outside, play, plant a garden, watch documentaries, find cool videos about health on Youtube, and make changes...*together!*

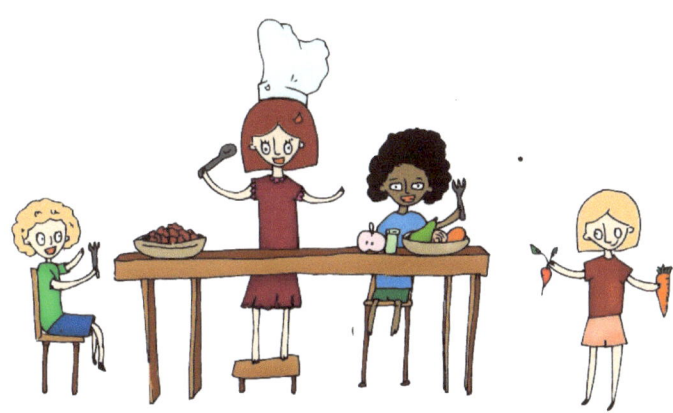

# Um...How about No?!

One of the next things you need to learn more about are GMOs and non-organic foods. Learning about this topic can be frustrating because non-organic and GMO foods are pretty much everywhere. There is really no escaping them. Learning about something that is bad for you but you are going to eat anyways doesn't feel very good. It almost feels like "well, what's the point?" But the reason we still have to learn about these foods is that even though we can't stop eating all non-organic, GMO foods by being more aware of their danger, we can at least eat **LESS** of them and *that of course is better than eating more*.

Non-organic plants are usually sprayed down with tons of artificial pesticides (bug spray) that help kill the bugs that eat them. But, when farmers spray plants with those chemicals and we eat the plants, their fruits and vegetables, or the animals that were fed those plants then, we too eat those harsh chemicals. Eating toxic bug killing chemicals is not cool.

The other bad part of non-organic foods is that when toxic chemicals are sprayed on the plants to keep bugs from eating them, the chemicals also fall on their flowers, nearby plants, in the water (streams and rivers), and the air. This then affects animals like the bees for example. The bees go from flower to flower and carry those chemicals back home to their hive. At the hive, the other bees become polluted with the chemicals, get sick, and die.

Bees are extremely important. Without bees, there is no pollination (what happens when bees go from one flower to flower). Without pollination, plants can't produce vegetables and fruits. This means NO FRUITS AND VEGETABLES ANYWHERE! If all the bees die off, humans wont even be able to exist. A farmer might think he is doing a good thing by spraying his crops with non-organic pesticides because they work so well but, as time passes by, he is hurting himself, the people he is selling food to, and the planet. Organically grown foods are treated without the same types of chemicals and are therefore better for the planet and the people who eat the plants of course (*that's us*).

And what's the deal with GMOs? GMOs stands for **G**enetically **M**odified **O**rganisms. Modify means to change. I'm still learning all the details of GMOs. But, I do know one key thing about them. GMOS seeds are seeds that companies add stuff to or change to make them *better*.

Here is the problem with that. Just like the food manufacturers adding chemicals to foods to make sales better for **them,** what's better for companies is not always what's best for **you** or your health. One example is when companies modify seeds so that they have pesticides inside them. Those seeds are now GMO seeds that then grow up into GMO plants that bugs wont eat. It's like spraying plants for bugs but from the inside out since the companies are putting the bug spray *inside* the seeds. If you are a farmer that's great for YOU because, you have less bugs eating up your plants. The problem is not for the farmer. The farmer is happy. The problem is for you and me who are eating the fruits and vegetables (or foods made with them) from those plants. If the seeds have bug spray so do those fruits and vegetables that grow from the seeds. That means you are eating BUG SPRAY with every bite! **Is eating bug spray is healthy**? Of course not!

Even though no one knows all of the dangers of eating foods made from GMOs if you can imagine eating a little bit of bug spray in every one of your meals every day for years, you can kind of figure out that at some point, all that bug spray is going to hurt you.

Adding pesticide is just one example of a change or modification that a company will make to a seed. There are other modifications. With each modification, there is a different risk. Over time, the risks add up. So even if we don't know all the details, we can probably agree that eating **less** GMOs is a good idea.

Talking to my mom helped me understand the dangers of pesticides and GMOs a little better. I also read The Omnivore's Dilemma: Young Readers Edition (I call it the Corn Book because it talked so much about corn) and watched the documentary **GMO OMG!** with her too. After reading and watching the documentary, my mother and I decided to buy foods that were non-GMO and organic foods whenever possible. We also eat less animal products (more about this in the meat section), buy more vegetables from local farmers (who use less GMOs seeds and pesticides), and to plant our own small garden once a year.

---

Watch **GMO OMG!** with your family or just learn more about GMOS and come up with your own family plan on how to reduce GMOs in your diet. **Then, as an added bonus make a video or post about it and share it on social media for others to learn.**

Use the internet to research why saving the bees is important and how we can all help do this very important task. You will be amazed at this issue and our part in it!

---

# Become an Ingredient Detective

By now, you are already starting to understand what types of things you shouldn't eat if you want to be healthy. In this section we will go over a few more details. Some of this stuff is a lot to keep up with at first but, the more you start thinking about these things and putting them into practice, the easier it all gets.

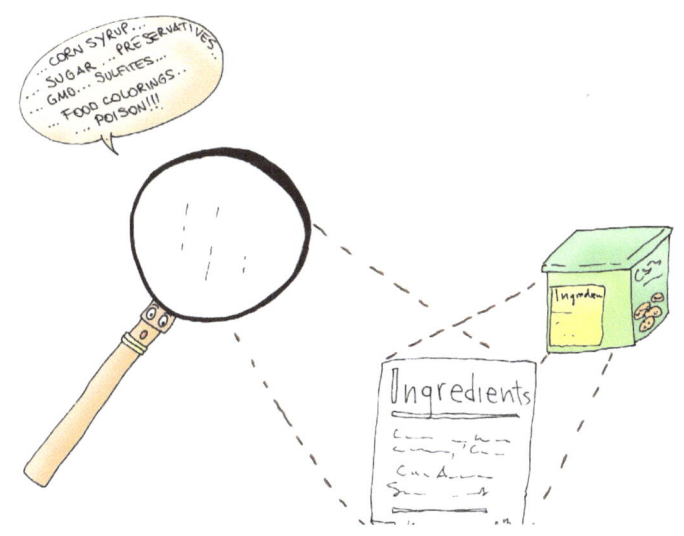

One thing you must get good at is to start looking at the ingredients of the foods you are eating. **Usually foods that have over 6-7 grams of sugar per serving have way too much sugar for you to process.** Sugar is harmful to your brain, gut, kidneys, and pancreas all at once.

When you look at a food label, also look at the SERVING SIZE of what you are eating. Start using the serving size to figure out if you are eating too much sugar or just too much of the food in general.

You might need an adult to walk you through this at first until you get the hang of it. Let's look take the example of toaster pastries.

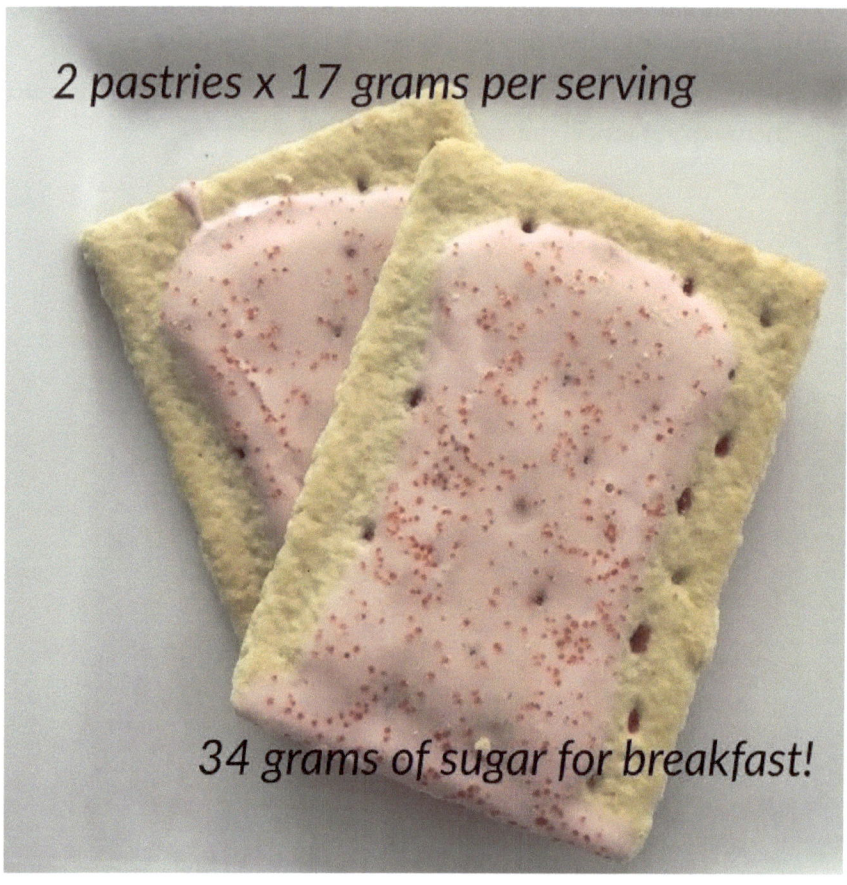

*2 pastries x 17 grams per serving*

*34 grams of sugar for breakfast!*

The label says that the serving size is ONE pastry and that it has 17g of sugar. Each pack in the box comes with two pastries not one. Most people would actually eat the two pastries in the pack. That means most people aren't eating 17g of sugar, they are actually eating 34 grams of sugar (17 x 2). To eat 34 grams of sugar in just ONE breakfast or snack is insane! That's just way too much sugar. But, it happens all the time because we aren't reading the labels in everything that we eat so we don't notice how much sugar we are actual eating.

In addition to sugar, keep an eye out for ingredients like **corn syrup, high fructose corn syrup, corn solids, soy, soy protein, corn, soy flour, and wheat.** Some people can handle eating wheat, corn, and soy products. You and your family will have to decide if that's the case for you. But, because these foods are usually grown with GMO seeds, making sure they are non-GMO is a must. And because they tend to be inflammatory eating LESS of them is usually good for everybody.

Common chemicals that are added to foods have names like **TBHQ, sulfites, BHA, BHT, glumate, glutamic acid, monosodium glutamate, magnesium glutamate, calcium glutamate, maltodextrin, sucralose, protein isolate, and funky colors with**

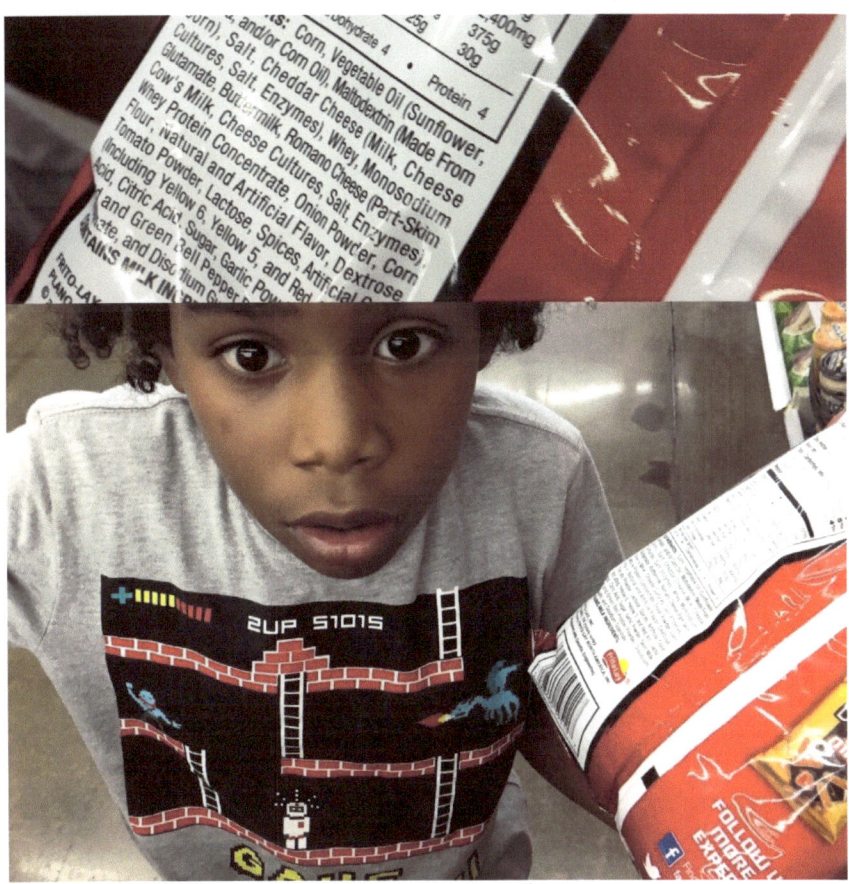

**numbers like red 3G and yellow 2G**. Again, these ingredients can damage your gut, your brain, and your clean up crew. They can even make you addicted to foods, affect your brain development (how it grows) AND influence your behavior by making you more hyper and unfocused. You don't want that! If the ingredients in the food sound entirely funky and artificial and they are really challenging to read, you probably want to say away from that food if you can.

Nitrates and nitrites are found in most hot dogs (in beef, chicken, and turkey ones too), bacon, and luncheon meats. These ingredients are

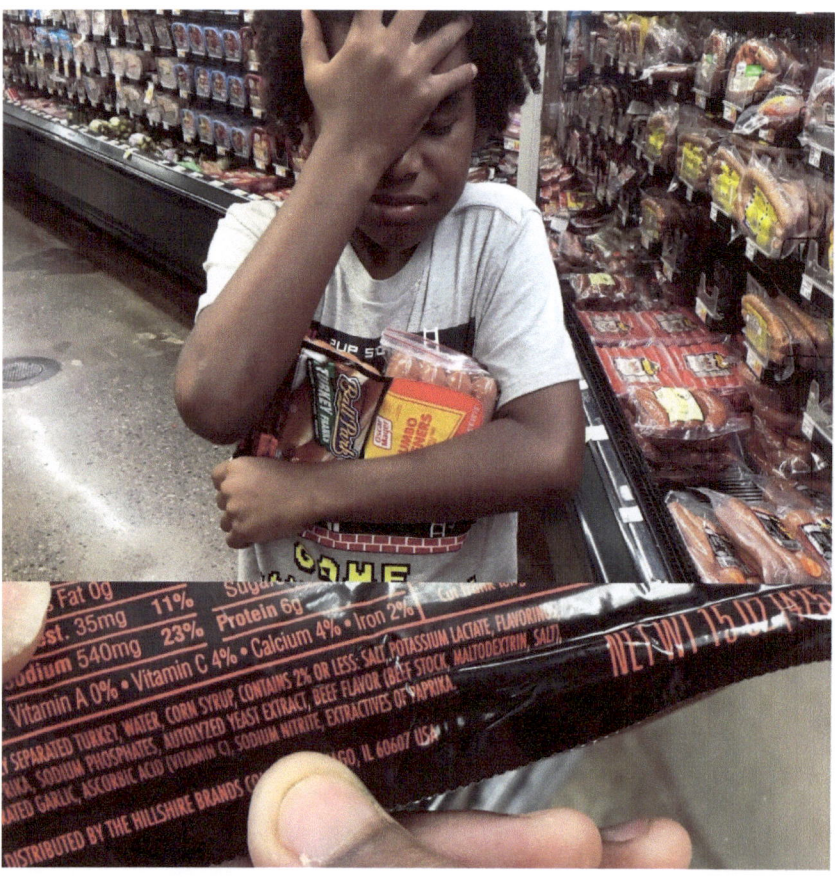

linked to cancer and kids. C-A-N-C-E-R! This is a serious disease. If your family is going to buy and eat processed meats, make sure you guys are picking nitrate-free ones. When you go to birthday parties or restaurants, where foods like hot dogs or luncheon meats are offered to kids, just say "no, thanks" and skip out because you don't know if are nitrate-free meats or not. Ask yourself, what's more important, protecting your health against a disease like cancer OR eating a hot dog or lunch sandwich?

Get into the habit of reading labels and ingredients **with** your family and your friends. The more everyone knows the easier it is for everybody. **When in doubt, just eat whole fruits and vegetables.**

---

**I found nitrates in at least 5 common brands of hot dogs!** Take a look at some of the ingredients in the foods you ate today (or have around your house). Do you see many of the damaging ingredients highlighted in this section?

---

## Water not juice and never soda

One of the fastest ways to start on your healthy lifestyle is to drink water, not juice, and never soda or sugar drinks like sports drinks and chocolate or strawberry milk! Think about it, if you want your plants to grow or a pet to stay healthy, what do you give them to drink? Water. You don't give them anything else. Why? Because all living things need clean $H_2O$ WATER to live. If you give them other things to drink, most plants and animals get sick, don't grow, and can even die over time. Humans are living things. We also need clean water to live. The organs in your body and the blood that flows through your veins are made of mostly water! They need water to work properly.

When you take an apple or an orange and you squeeze them to make juice out of it, their juice still has all the nutrients and enzymes of that fruit. That's good. But, if you leave that juice out on the counter or even in the refrigerator for more than a few days, it dies, then it goes bad.

The food manufacturers have to make juice that doesn't go bad because it's going to go to the store and sit on the shelves and in your house for a long time. In order to do that, they have to do something to the juice that kills the fruits' healthy enzymes. This processes is called pasteurization. Without the enzymes of the fruit, even 100% juice is mostly sugar and doesn't have all the nutrients of fruit.

40

Excess sugar shrinks your brain, makes your body acidic, triggers inflammation and mucus, and throws off your gut, kidneys, and pancreas. Artificial chemicals and additives in other drinks tax your clean up crew. Non-juice drinks like soda and fruit punch are full of sugar and chemicals. As good as they taste, drinking them is not a good idea. It is hurtful.

Next time you go to drink anything other than water look at the ingredients. How many grams of sugar are in that one drink? How many chemicals and colors in the ingredients? You will soon start to see how much sugar and added stuff you are drinking. Water should be your daily go-to drink. It is what your body is made of and what you need.

## Toxins OUT not ON!

Remember how your skin is a protective shield that keeps toxins out? Well, eating your toxins isn't good but neither is putting them right on your skin. If you use products like shampoo, toothpaste, conditioner, lotion, soap, and bug spray with lots of chemicals then they go right through you skin and into your bloodstream.

Some chemicals found in shampoos, lotions, and other products have been linked to SERIOUS diseases from asthma to Alzheimers and cancer. This doesn't mean that if you use regular shampoo or bug spray one time you will get sick. But, that using toxic products every day of your life is impacting your organs and stressing your cleaning crew. Over time, this can have real negative consequences.

When you are looking through the ingredients on products these are some of names you want to avoid: **parabens, polyethylene glycol (PEG), sodium laureth sulfate (Sles), sodium lauryl sulfate (Sls), formaldehyde, quaternium-15, DMDM hydantoin, imidazolidinyl urea, diazolidinyl urea, polyoxymethylene urea, sodium hydroxymethylglycinate, 2-bromo-2-nitropropane-1,3-diol (bromopol) and glyoxal.**

These names are insane, right? You wouldn't eat these ingredients. Clearly, they are chemicals. Then, don't put them on your body. They will enter your bloodstream just the same!

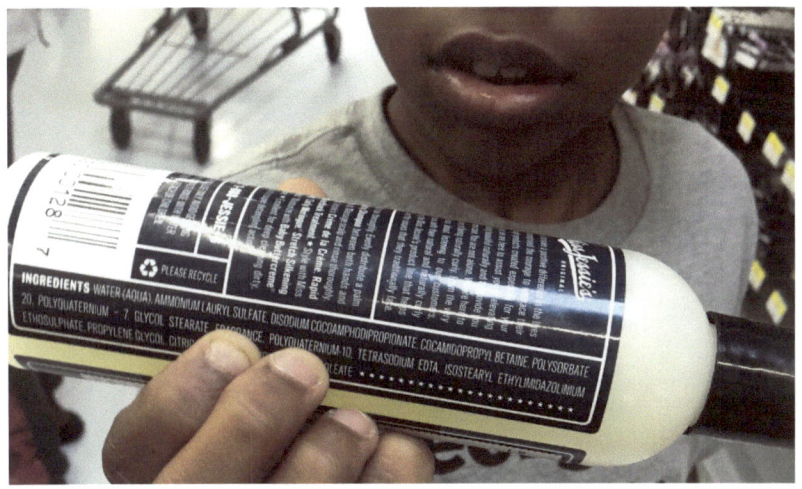

*My mom was just about to buy this shampoo one day and I saw that she didn't turn it around and look at the label. I asked her to and BOOM, what did we find? Sulfates! We didn't buy it of course.*

And as far as bug spray goes, stay away from products made with **DEET.** There are tons of other bug sprays made without it. Sure you don't want to get bitten by mosquitos, but DEET is extremely toxic and it affects children the most! Protect your brain. Protect your cells.

The best way to defend ourselves against toxicity is to avoid or prevent it. This means that whenever possible, it's important to use products that are natural and don't have lots of chemicals and toxins (specially those already linked to diseases). Read the labels of your foods *and* your products with your parents and with your friends. Try to stick to products that don't have lots of toxicity like plain castille soap, coconut oil, shea butter, fluoride-free toothpaste, and natural bug spray without DEET. Those are usually better choices.

## Meat or No Meat?

You may have noticed a lot more people and some of your friends talking about going or being vegan or vegetarian. Vegetarians don't eat meat but, do eat other foods that come from animals like honey, milk, yogurt, cheese, and eggs. Vegans don't eat any foods that come from animals at all.

Depending on what your family believes or what you may know about health you may or may not believe that eating meat and other animal products is healthy or unhealthy. Some people say "yes, eating animal products is good for you" and other people say "no eating animal products is bad for you don't eat them." How each family feels or even each person within the family will be different.

The thing about eating meat is that *well*...it comes from animals and you might not have thought about it but, that means that animals have to die for you to get their meat. To a lot of people, kids included, that doesn't sound or feel good once you put some thought into it because animals are living things. You and your family might be okay with that. That doesn't make you a bad person and doesn't necessarily mean you are unhealthy either. But, it is something to think about.

Meat and dairy can also be acidic and most dairy (milk, cheese, and yogurt) in particular is mucus forming and inflammatory to your gut. Oh, and remember those GMOs we talked about? Most animals eat food that's made from GMOs. If the animals eat them, and we eat the animals, in an indirect way we are also eating those GMOS.

Also, because animals are raised not in beautiful farms like you see in cartoons or in commercials but in crowded, crammed spaces, they end up eating, living, sleeping, and using the bathroom all in the same space. Imagine sleeping, eating, and going to bathroom all in same space with hundreds of other animals doing the same thing. What do you think happens? <Hint: why do we wash our hands when we use the bathroom?> You probably guessed right. The animals get sick a lot and have to be given medicine. If the animals are given medicine and then we eat the animals then it's like we are taking the medicine too.

In general taking medicine can be good for us IF we are sick. But, think about it. Is it healthy to take medicine for no reason? No. It can actually be very harmful and dangerous. Taking medicine when not needed stresses your clean up crew PLUS causes inflammation in your gut. Is this good? Of course not. So even if you don't believe eating animals or animal products is unhealthy, you can at least see that because animals are raised eating GMOS and then given medicines to treat diseases, their meat is probably not the healthiest you can eat. *By the way, I learned a lot about this the "corn book" I mentioned before. It's really a good book to read with your parents.*

Lastly, because people eat so much meat, raising animals for meat and for dairy takes up a LOT of space, energy, and water (for the animals to drink and also to clean up all the waste <poop>). So does growing all the GMO plants for them to eat! Trees have to be cut to make room for this space. Less trees and wasted energy and water is bad for the earth. *We all know that.*

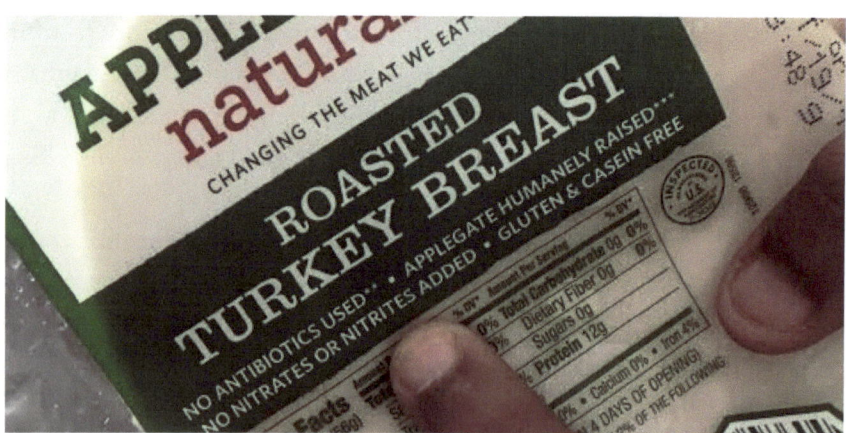

If you and your family still do want to eat meat and animals products, look for key words like NO hormones, humanely raised, NO nitrates or nitrites, NO antibiotics, and casein free. And, try to eat non-GMO, organic, pastured meat, dairy, and eggs instead of regular ones. Pastured means the animals are eating grass instead of animal feed made with wheat, soy, corn, and/or other animals. It usually also means the animals are being raised in kinder environments.

You should also try to eat the least processed, more natural versions of any animal products you do eat. So for example, if you are using honey, try using raw honey. If you are eating chicken, eat a piece of chicken instead of a chicken nugget. If you are wanting to eat an egg sandwich, having your mom make one with fresh pastured eggs, whole grain bread, and goat or organic raw cheese is going to be a better option than eating a frozen or fast food egg sandwich with a zillion chemicals on it. Makes sense? Less processed, more humane, less chemicals.

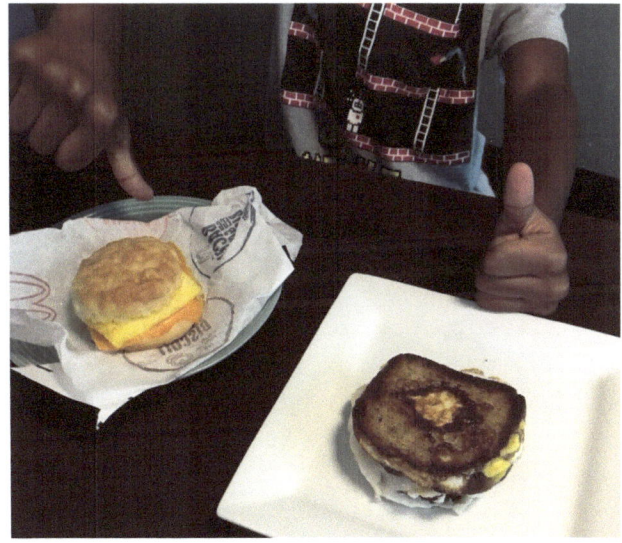

In the end, whether you eat no meat or animal products or if you do, **eating at least less of them**, means less animals have to die, there is less waste of land, energy, and water created and you'll end up with less GMOs and random medicine on your plate. Eating less meat and animal products also gives you a chance to eat more vegetables and fruits. That's a good deal, right?

It is important to know that all people whether they eat meat, some animal products, or no animal products can be committed to being healthy and be respectful of each other. Never make fun of what people eat or be mean to someone because of what they or their family eats.

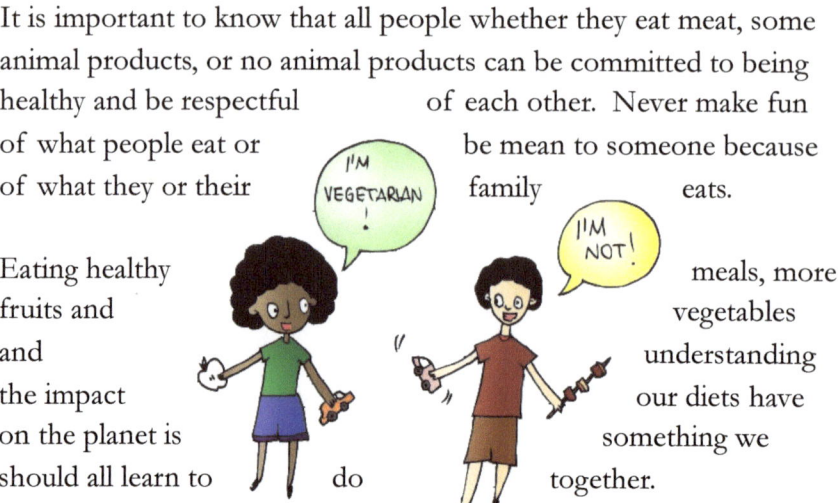

Eating healthy fruits and vegetables and understanding the impact our diets have on the planet is something we should all learn to do together.

If you and your family are interested in becoming a vegan or a vegetarian and would like to watch two "kid-friendly" videos. Search the following titles on youtube:

1.) 5 Reasons We Don't Eat Meat! [For Kids!]
2.) KIDS! Just Say No to MILK [For Kids]

# Move Your Body & Get Outside

Your body needs exercise for many reasons. It makes your heart and muscles strong and it keeps your weight balanced. But, it does more than that. Exercise also helps your body detox and reduce stress.

How exactly does exercise do that? One is that when you exercise you start to sweat and sweat releases waste through your skin (*helloooo* clean up crew). Another way is also by helping what is called the lymphatic system.

If you know anything about what a city's sewer system does, you know it is VERY important to keeping a city clean and healthy. A sewer system connects to every single house and building through a network of pipes and tunnels. It then takes **all** of their the sinks', showers', and toilets' **dirty** water away from those houses and buildings and into a special place to get processed and cleaned because, well…dirty water is **nasty** and we need clean water to live.

Your lymphatic system. It is a (like pipes) that throughout moments of the the waste in your the system that antibodies (the diseases) in your

system is your body's own sewer system of vessels is connected all your body, at all day, and gets rid of organs. It ALSO is creates and delivers stuff that fights body.

Movement is kind of like *flushing the toilet or running your faucet.* Flushing your toilet after using the bathroom is a good idea. It gets the dirty water out and it gets the new clean water in for next time. The same thing with running your sink. Doing these things are both giving you something (clean water) and taking something away (dirty water). This is exactly how movement and exercise work. When you move you help your lymphatic system pump those dirty fluids **out** and get the antibodies **in.** You need flow to get fluids to GO!

Also, if you remember hormones are what regulate stress. Too much stress means excess inflammation. Exercise and movement help the body regulate stress hormones. Less stress means less inflammation. This is good, right? By now you know the answer: of course.

Finally, when you are moving, playing, exercising, or just plain going **outside**, you also absorb the sunlight through your skin which gives you vitamin D. Vitamin D makes your bones strong, fights diseases, and puts you in a better mood. Can it get any better?

# A Healthy Mind

Believe it or not, being healthy is not just about eating good foods, avoiding bad foods and skin products, getting good rest, drinking water, and moving our bodies. There is one more thing we need to think about and that is having a healthy mind. The mind is the place where your thoughts live. Your thoughts and your body are connected. If your mind is always thinking of negative things it will eventually make your body sick. *It also makes you not so fun to be around.*

You give your body good healthy foods to keep it healthy. Positive thoughts are like health food for your mind. In order to have a healthy mind, you have to feed it positive thoughts.

Start paying attention to the things you tell yourself and the attitude that you have about things. Do you say things like this all the time?

- "I'm bored. This is boring."
- "I'm stupid. This is stupid."
- "I'm not good at things."
- "I hate this."
- "I don't care."
- "I'm ugly. That person is ugly."
- "I don't matter."
- "I hate my hair."
- "No one likes me."

Saying those kinds of things will have you having an unhealthy mind. They are the junk food of thoughts. Instead choose to feed yourself positive thoughts every day. Here are some examples:

- "I am open to new things."
- "I am an important member of my family."
- "I am a good person."

- "I can do anything I put my mind to."
- "I am a great friend."
- "I make friends easily."
- "I love myself."
- "I care about my life."
- "I find the good in things."

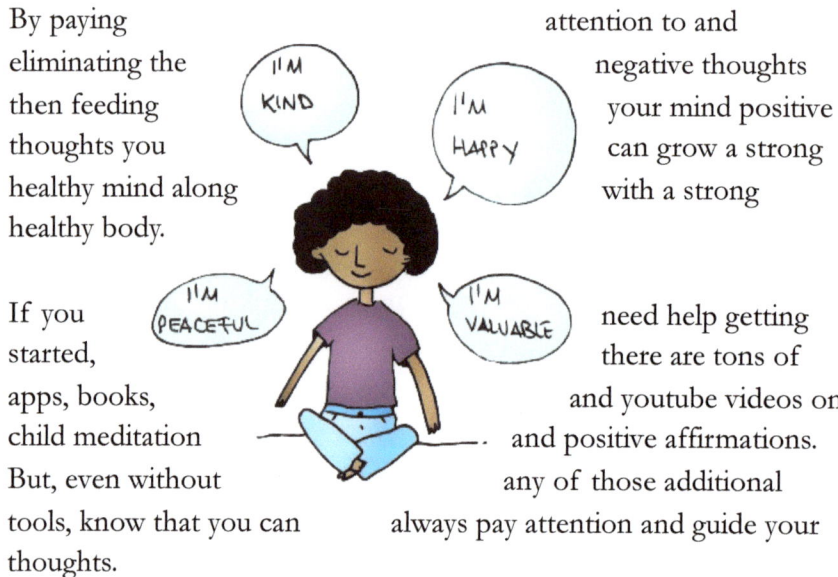

By paying attention to and eliminating the negative thoughts then feeding your mind positive thoughts you can grow a strong healthy mind along with a strong healthy body.

If you need help getting started, there are tons of apps, books, and youtube videos on child meditation and positive affirmations. But, even without any of those additional tools, know that you can always pay attention and guide your thoughts.

# From Healthy Kid to Healthy Person

Think about what you have read so far. It might feel like it's a lot to learn but it really isn't once you start putting it all into practice. The most important thing you have to remember is that **your body is valuable**.

It is really, really smart and has incredible organs and systems that work for you around the clock. All you have to do is to take care of them and they will take care of you. They actually WANT to take care of you! They just need a little help.

How you take care of them is by keeping toxins out, nutrients in, moving around, getting sunshine, resting up, drinking water, and feeding your mind good thoughts. This is also how you show your friends and the world that you love yourself. In order to that, there are a few things you need to do but they are all easy. Let's review some of the things we have learned about in this guide:

- Learn to read labels on all your foods AND the products you use on your skin.
- Look out for ingredient labels that list a bunch of chemicals. Some chemicals like MSG (**monosodium glutamate) and parabens (in shampoos and lotions)** should be on your OH NO radar!
- If it doesn't say NON-GMO then the food was made with GMO. Try to stay away or eat less of these foods.
- Use non-chemical toothpaste, lotion, soap, shampoo, and conditioner.
- Watch out for serving size. Learn to figure out what serving size and sugar amount you are *really* eating. This a great way to practice math.

- Eat mostly fruit and vegetables as a part of your diet and less processed foods. This includes processed animal products and meats, if you and your family are not vegetarians or vegans.
- Drink water. Sodas, fruit drinks, and juices are not what your body needs.
- Practice saying "no" to junk foods. The more you do it, the easier it gets.
- Go outside. Movement and sunshine are great for you.
- Too much screen time (video games, tablets, tv) and not enough sleep increases stress. Work with your parents to find a balance.
- Feed your mind positive thoughts and stay away from negative ones.

These are all things you can actually do. You just have to get started and practice. Begin to do these things EVERY DAY as a child and do them for the rest of your life. These are the things that will keep you and your family healthy.

Stay away from fast foods, sugar cereals, candies, chips, cookies, nuggets, boxed mac and cheese…*you know "kid" foods*. Eat REAL food instead.

Even when your family makes changes inside your home, outside the world will always be full of junkie foods. You have to be prepared to make good choices for yourself. When visiting friends and family that don't have healthy options, be polite and just say "no thanks." You don't have to feel bad for saying "no" or tell them *their* food is not healthy (that's rude), just care about your health enough to stick to what you believe in. Play with and love them just the same.

Birthday parties and play dates can be extra tricky. My mom usually packs something for me and makes sure I eat before I leave the house so I won't be starrrrrrvvviiing and really wanting to dig into food I normally wouldn't eat. **This is something we pretty much do every day. It is a great family practice.** When it's time to eat, I just eat my packed food and snacks.

Something else I do at parties and play dates is see what options I have, including the non-healthy ones. If there is something that I really want to eat, I eat that ONE thing. Of course, I'm not going to pick something too unhealthy like soda or chips with MSG (like Doritos or Takis) and I try not to pick the ice cream because it has dairy and sugar but, I may pick from the 100% juice box, a cookie, plain chips, or *say*, a popsicle. Whatever I choose, I eat one serving of that one thing. This lets me eat a little bit of party stuff without totally junking up my body.

Having to make tough choices is when sharing information and learning with friends and family comes in handy. The more we all learn together, the less junky foods and more healthy foods we will have in each other's homes and parties. This makes life so much easier.

Your decisions today affect your future. Choose health. Be a healthy kid now and later, a healthy adult. You can do it.

## Ideas for Healthy Meals

My mom and I have worked on a list of foods and snack ideas which are healthy and kid-friendly. Because everyone's family is different, we included vegan and vegetarian ideas but also some that are not. Check them out below. Soon I will be posting videos and recipes with my mom on youtube. Check out www.youtube.com/urbanbailout and look for the Nicholas' Health Videos Playlist.

### Breakfast ideas

- Plain oatmeal (add honey/ maple syrup/dates to sweeten and top with nuts, raisins, or fresh fruit like apples or bananas)
- Low sugar sugar gluten free cereal with almond or coconut milk
- Fruit or green smoothie
- Plain fruit
- Fruit and almond butter
- Tofu

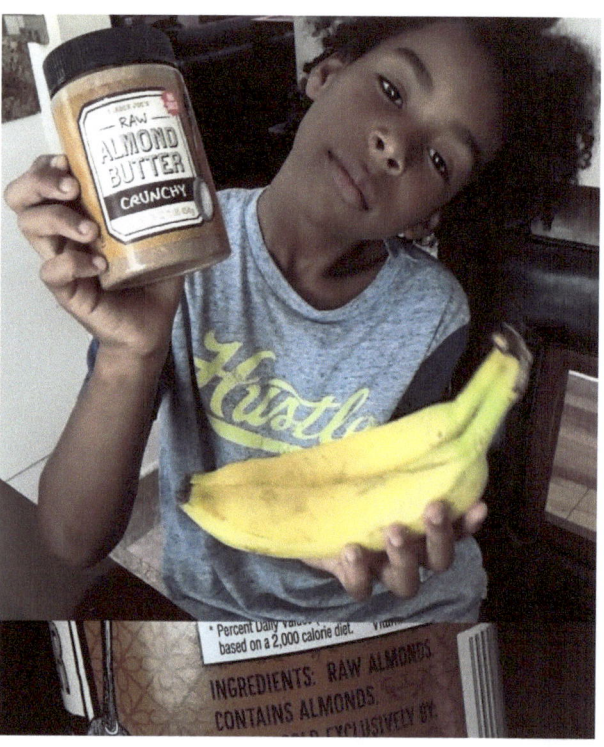

Find nut and seed butters that do not have added sugar and oils. This almond butter has only one ingredient: almonds.

scramble with vegetables and gluten free toast
- Buckwheat pancakes with real maple syrup (not pancake syrup)
- French toast using gluten free whole grain bread with real maple syrup (can be made vegan style - without eggs)
- Non-vegan option: Egg and gluten free toast or scrambled eggs and vegetables topped with salsa or low sugar ketchup

*Gluten free bread is just an option. Non-GMO whole grain spelt or wheat might work for you too. When eating tofu, look for NON-GMO, organic versions.

### ~Lunch and dinner ideas
- Almond or peanut butter and raw honey, natural fruit spread, or banana sandwich with gluten free whole grain bread. If your school doesn't allow nuts or if you are allergic you can try sunflower butter and add maple syrup to make sunflower a little sweeter.
- Fruit or green smoothie (freeze overnight then put in a thermos to defrost if you are packing a lunch)
- Homemade cheese quesadilla or mini pizza (vegan or organic cheese, add a few vegetables, use bread slices or tortillas as your pizza crust and then add sauce and toppings)

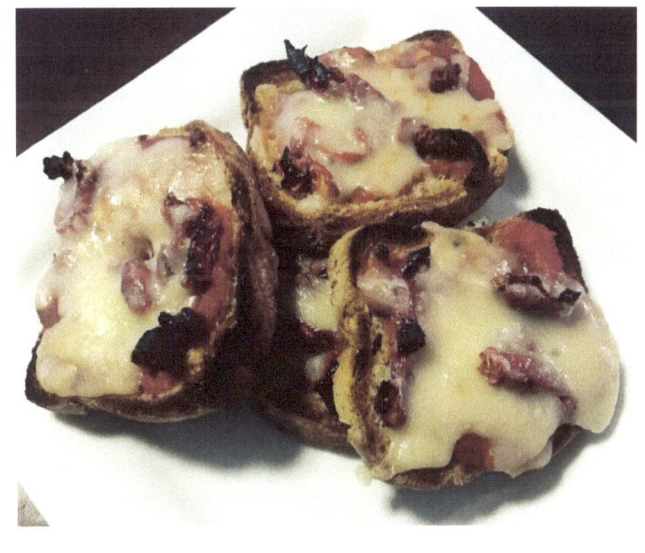

- Black bean dip tortilla chips (non-

57

gmo) and/ or salsa and a side of fruit (like sliced apples, tangerine, banana)

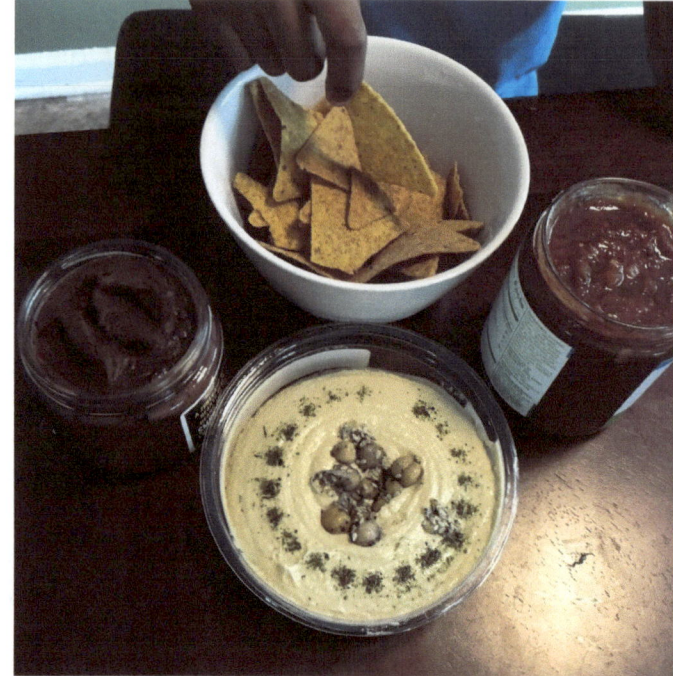

- Hummus and pita bread or humus sandwich with gluten free bread and a side of fruit
- Soups! Homemade tomato, black bean, butternut squash, and lentil soups are my favorite. Store bought soup in a BPA free carton or BPA free can, preferably organic.
- Pasta salad or pasta and marinara (red) sauce, no meat needed. Vegetables can be added is a bonus. If you don't love vegetables, an adult can puree some in blender and add to the sauce. You won't even taste them!
- Rice and beans with a vegetable as side (my favorite sides are avocado or cabbage)
- Burritos or tacos (rice, beans, salsa, non-gmo or pastured meat, and vegan cheese <optional>).
- Sauteed mushrooms (I looooove mushrooms) with your favorite vegetable) and brown rice
- Vegetable stir fry and rice or quinoa
- Find a vegetable (or a few of them) that you like and eat a lot of them!

- Turkey rollups (nitrate-free turkey) with or without pita bread or a sandwich. Try vegan cheese, organic cheese, or even better no cheese at all.
- Boiled eggs (pastured)
- Chicken kabob (*or fried non-gmo organic tofu*) and homemade baked french fries or sweet potato fries

**~Snacks and desserts**

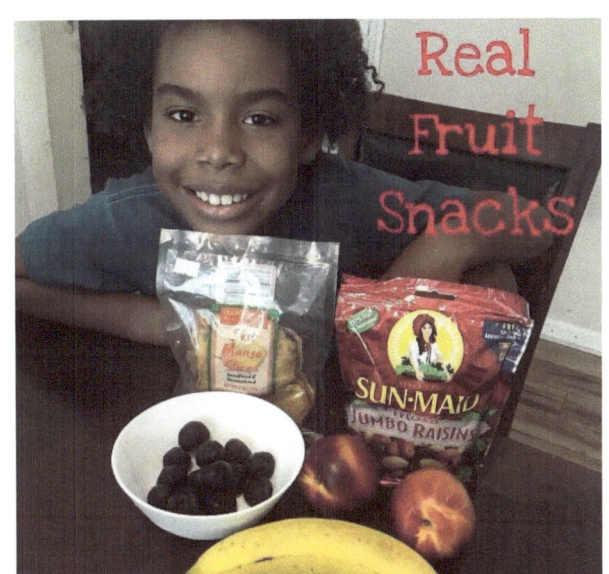

- Fruit (not fruit cups), fresh, frozen, or dried (I LOVE frozen cherries, frozen grapes, and dried mangoes)
- Homemade organic non-gmo granola bars (low on the sugar)
- Lara bars (the kind at stores or homemade)
- Healthy banana cookies (have an adult find some recipes on Google. I make them with my mom with just bananas, gluten free oatmeal, peanut butter, and nuts or vegan chocolate chips or raisins)
- Gluten free corn chips and salsa and/or guacamole or black bean dip (it took me a while to like these dips but I LOVE them now!)
- Non-GMO popcorn
- Homemade low sugar muffins with some vegetable purees mixed in. Great book for parents: Sneaky Chef.
- Date rolls (I like the kind with coconut) or dates and almond butter or peanut butter

- Trail mix (I like Trader Joe's raw trail mix)
- Healthy soft serve ice cream (it's make made with frozen bananas not milk. Have an adult find recipes on the internet)
- Healthy "milk" shake (coconut or almond milk, ice cubes, dates, almond butter, and vanilla - YUM!)
- Plain coconut yogurt or goat kefir with maple syrup or raw honey and fresh fruit

*You can also use fruit as a default. A little fruit is a snack, a little more is a meal.*

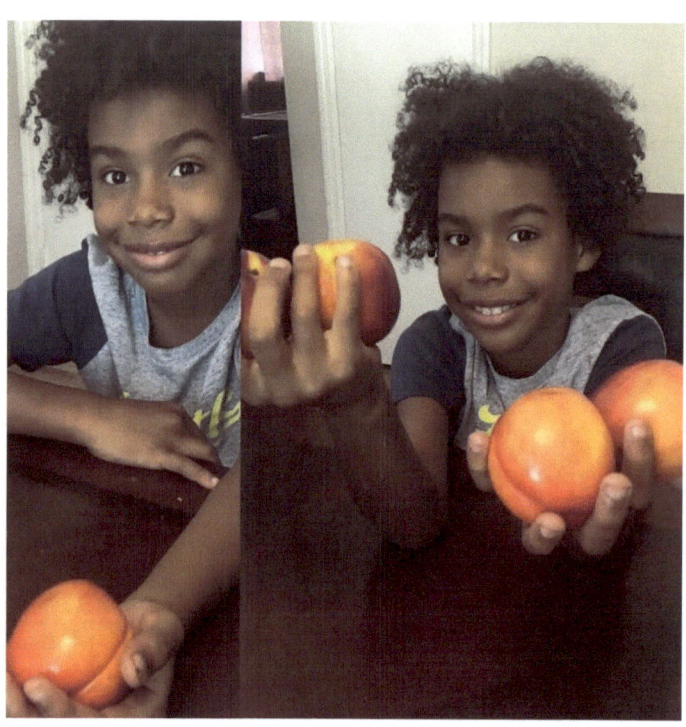

# Just a Kid, Huh?

I'm sure at some point while you were reading this book or even in your life you have thought to yourself "But I'm just a kid. I can't change the way I eat. I can't change things in my life. My parents buy my food. My parents control my life." In some ways you are right, sometimes you do have to do what your parents (or other adults) tell you and eat what they give you. I totally get that. But, what you have to understand that is the YOU DO HAVE POWER over your life and lots of influence.

For starters, you always have control over what you think, what you tell yourself, and what you choose to believe. Feed you mind positive thoughts. Eliminate negative thoughts. That part is entirely up to you. As you get older, and if you have access to the internet, you have more control of what you learn. Use the internet to learn about your body, your health, meditation, exercise, and healthy foods that you eat. You also have access to books at the public or school library.

Think about it, when a new video game or toy comes out, children of all ages find ways to learn all about them. Kids are master investigators! One day I knew nothing about Minecraft. A few months later, I knew everything about it! How? It was what I wanted to do. I found ways to research. I found videos. I asked my friends. I begged my mom for Minecraft books. That's just what we do. We are great at it. Use that same skill and energy and put it into learning more about your health.

Kids also have lots of influence over our parents, other adults, and our friends. We just don't realize it. That's exactly why toy makers and food manufacturers make commercials just for US. Restaurants have kid's menus just for US. Supermarkets have entire isles of foods designed just for US. Think about all the kid's cereals at the grocery store. Those cereals are made mostly for US. Clearly, we have influence.

A lot of the things you have, the movies you watch, the songs you listen to, the toys you play with, and yes, the foods you eat, even the junky ones, you have picked or at least, have had some say over it. Your parents get you nuggets, cookies, and breakfast muffins because you have asked for them or because you have said that you like them. Your friends might always play video games at your house because that's what you always suggest. But, there is nothing stopping you from suggesting an outdoor game or more physical activity, for you to talk to your friends and family about making healthier choices, or for you to ask for more healthy foods at the grocery store. **You use your voice all the time. Start using it for change.**

Begin by asking and saying the right things to your parents (*in a polite way*). Here are some examples:

- "Do you think it's okay if we switch our milk to almond milk?"
- "Can we use a shampoo with less chemicals?"
- "Would it be okay if I took off the pepperoni or the cheese from this pizza and just ate the crust with sauce?"
- "I read the kid's versions of these foods have more sugar and chemicals. Would you mind if we get plain oatmeal and just add honey and bananas instead of getting this kind?"
- "No thank you. I will just have water please."
- "Can we stop and get some apples and bananas at the supermarket instead of a happy meal for lunch? It will cost the same."

Make sure that when they get you healthier things, you say "thank you" and that you eat them even if they aren't *as* tasty. Stay committed to being your best healthiest self!

There are also special times like birthdays, holidays, or a good report card when parents and other adults ask kids *specifically* "what do you want?" Use these times to ask for one meatless meal a week, no soda or juice at the party *(I know, I know, it's hard)*, or ask for your parents to watch a health documentary with you. Show your parents, adults, and friends that your health matters to you. Be helpful. Be polite. Use your power.

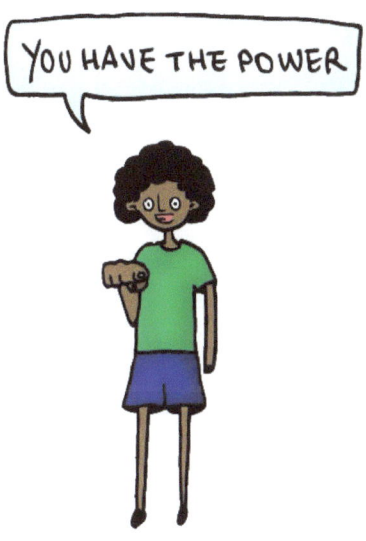

## Last Thoughts

I hope you liked my health guide and that you learned a lot. There are a lot of people, both children and adults, suffering from bad health today. The planet and the bees are also hurting because making these junk foods and GMOs are destroying life all over the world. It is important that we share the things we learn about health together. The more we learn and share the healthier we will be, so *share away*!

I will making more videos, guides, and posts (on instagram @outofthemouthofbabes and youtube.com/urbanbailout Nicholas' Health Videos Playlist). If you liked my book or have questions you want to ask me, you can email me through my mom's email account urbanbailout@gmail.com and put FOR NICHOLAS in the heading. I would love to hear more form you.

Stay healthy. Stay in touch! Thank you.

www.ingramcontent.com/pod-product-compliance
Lightning Source LLC
Chambersburg PA
CBHW050811290526
45792CB00001B/77